Eating Vegetarian

Easy & Tasty Recipes For Living And Eating Well Everyday

Brigitte S. Romeo

Eating Vegetarian

© **Copyright 2021 - All rights reserved.**

The content contained within this book may not be reproduced, duplicated or transmitted without direct written permission from the author or the publisher.

Under no circumstances will any blame or legal responsibility be held against the publisher, or author, for any damages, reparation, or monetary loss due to the information contained within this book. Either directly or indirectly.

Legal Notice:

This book is copyright protected. This book is only for personal use. You cannot amend, distribute, sell, use, quote or paraphrase any part, or the content within this book, without the consent of the author or publisher.

Disclaimer Notice:

Please note the information contained within this document is for educational and entertainment purposes only. All effort has been executed to present accurate, up to date, and reliable, complete information. No warranties of any kind are declared or implied. Readers acknowledge that the author is not engaging in the rendering of legal, financial, medical or professional advice. The content within this book has been derived from various sources. Please consult a licensed professional before attempting any techniques outlined in this book.

By reading this document, the reader agrees that under no circumstances is the author responsible for any losses, direct or indirect, which are incurred as a result of the use of information contained within this document, including, but not limited to, errors, omissions, or inaccuracies.

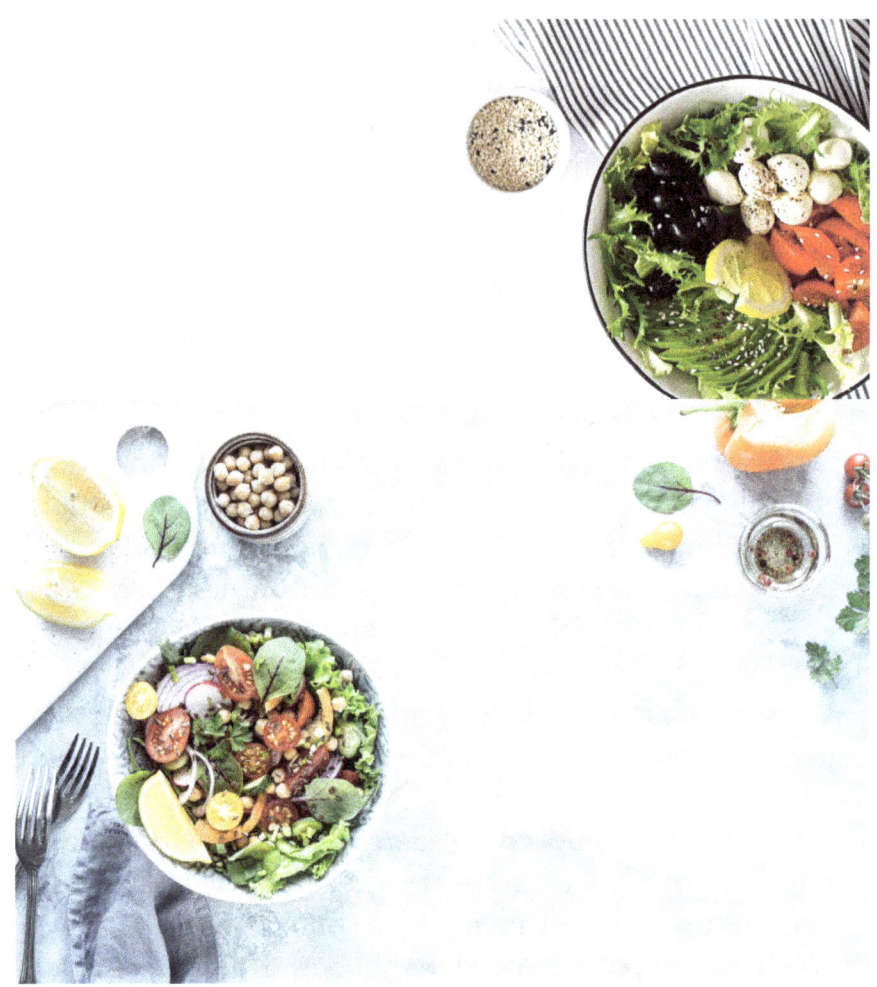

TABLE OF CONTENTS

INTRODUCTION **8**

CHAPTER 1: BREAKFAST RECIPES **10**

1. Amazing Almond & Banana Granola 10
2. Perfect Polenta with a Dose of Cranberries & Pears 13
3. Tempeh Bacon Smoked to Perfection 15
4. Vegan Muffins Breakfast Sandwich 17
5. Toasted Rye with Pumpkin Seed Butter 19
6. Overnight Oats 21
7. Chickpeas Spread Sourdough Toast 22

CHAPTER 2: LUNCH RECIPES **24**

8. Tomato Soup 24
9. Black Bean Soup 27
10. French Onion Soup 29

CHAPTER 3: MAIN MEALS RECIPES **32**

11. Stir Fry 32
12. Spanakorizo 34
13. Roast Chili Lime Chickpeas 36
14. Miso Spaghetti Squash 37

CHAPTER 4: VEGETABLES, SALADS AND SIDES RECIPES **40**

15. Mashed Cauliflower 40
16. Broccoli with Ginger and Garlic 42
17. Balsamic Roasted Carrots 43
18. Chives and Radishes Platter 44
19. Healthy Rosemary and Celery Dish 45
20. Hearty Cheesy Cauliflower 47

21.	Mesmerizing Spinach Quiche	48
22.	Simple Mushroom Hats and Eggs	50

CHAPTER 5: DESSERT RECIPES 52

23.	Salted Caramel Coconut Balls	52
24.	Baked Pears	54
25.	Chocolate Mousse	55
26.	Super Tea Spiced Poached Pears	57
27.	Warming Baked Apples	59

CHAPTER 6: SNACK RECIPES 62

28.	Lemon and Olive Pasta	62
29.	Cheesy Macaroni	65
30.	Creamy Mushroom Rigatoni	67
31.	Southwest Pasta	69
32.	Peanut Noodles	71
33.	Red Curry Noodles	73
34.	Sun-Dried Tomato Pasta	75

CHAPTER 7: JUICES AND SMOOTHIES RECIPES 78

35.	Beet and Orange Smoothie	78
36.	Strawberry, Banana, and Coconut Shake	80
37.	Green Colada	81
38.	Avocado Spinach Smoothie	82
39.	Almond Spinach Smoothie	83
40.	3-Ingredient Mango Smoothie	84

CHAPTER 8: OTHER RECIPES 86

41.	Tahini Miso Dressing	86
42.	Balsamic Roasted Tomatoes	88
43.	Crispy Spicy Chickpeas	90

44.	Roasted Pumpkin Seeds	92
45.	Lemony Breadcrumbs	93
46.	Cauliflower Skillet Steaks	95
47.	Lemony Kale, Avocado, And Chickpea Salad	97
48.	Lentil Potato Salad	99
49.	Curried Apple Chips	101
50.	Bok Choy–Asparagus Salad	103

CONCLUSION **104**

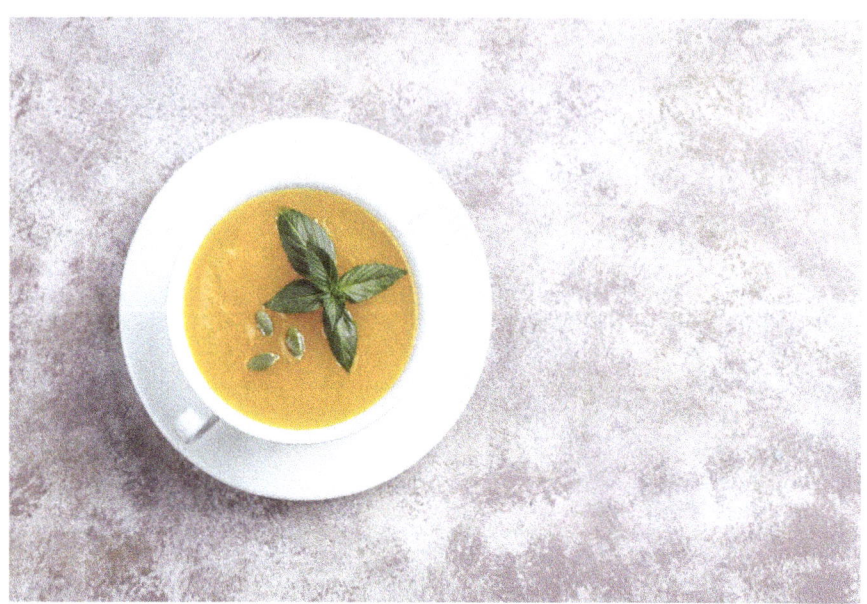
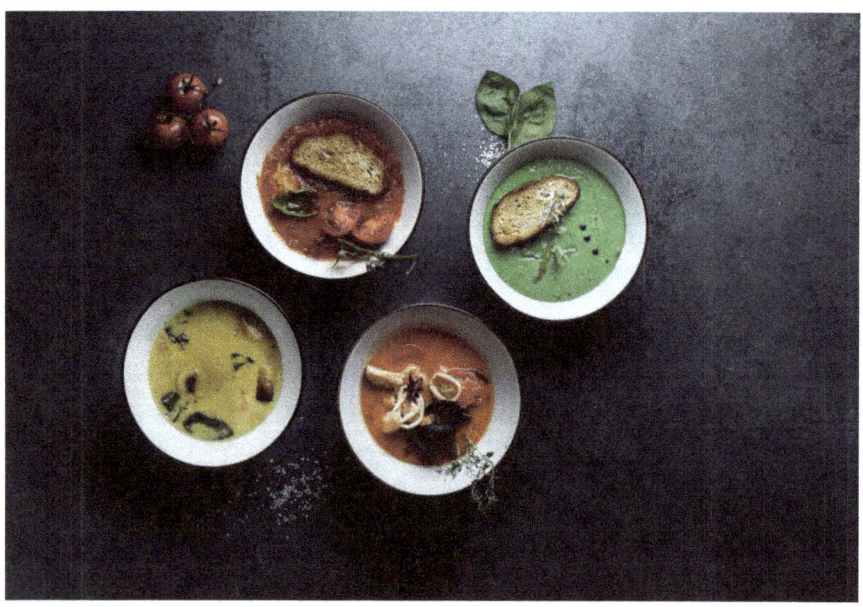

INTRODUCTION

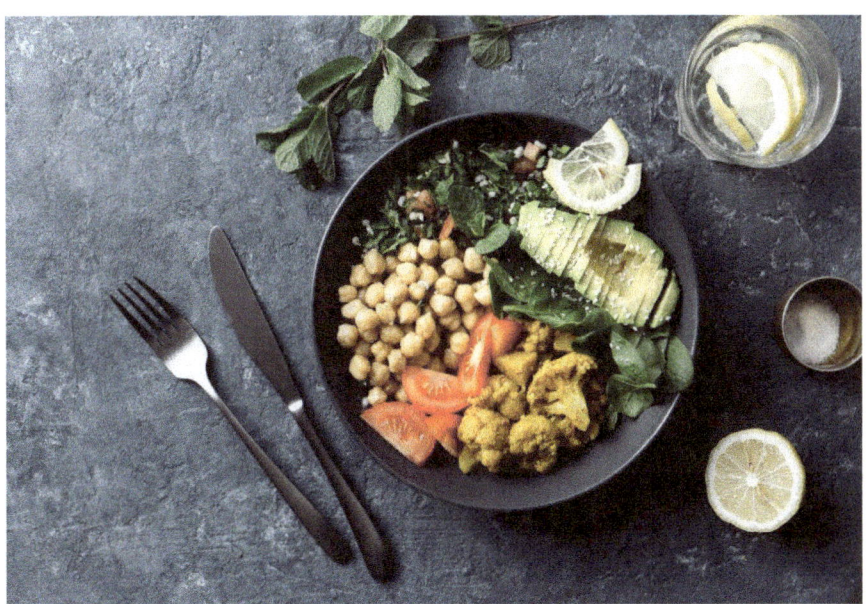

What does it mean to be a vegetarian?

Vegetarian is a person who does not eat meat, poultry, or fish. Vegetarians eat only plant foods such as fruits, vegetables, legumes, and grains or products made from them. Some people think of a vegetarian as a person who does not eat red meat but may consume fish and chicken. Other people consider a vegetarian to be someone who avoids eating all animal flesh, including fish, poultry, and red meat. However, "true" vegetarians avoid the consumption of all meats, including fish and chicken.

Vegetarianism is not a new concept; it has been practiced since ancient times in India during the Vedic period (1500-500 BC) as well as in Greece and Rome. It continues to be practiced today in modern society around the world. In most cases, it is a matter of individual choice.

Eating meat and fish has been a common practice all over the world for thousands of years. In some cultures, the preparation of the meat or fish symbolizes wealth and luxury, while in others it represents a source of survival. Today, people are becoming more aware of the impact that their food choices have on their health as well as on the environment.

Why do people become vegetarians? The reasons vary widely from person to person. Some people object to the cruelty and suffering of animals raised for food. Some people object to the environmental effects of producing meat and fish. Others become vegetarians because they believe animal flesh is unhealthy to eat or because they believe it is unspiritual or unwise. For some, it is a choice of economic necessity.

How often should you eat fruits and vegetables? The recommendation is to eat five servings per day based on a 2,000 calorie diet. One serving is equal to one-half cup raw or one cup ready-to-eat. Fruits and vegetables provide vitamins, minerals, fiber, and other nutrients that are essential for good health. It is recommended that most Americans make fruits and vegetables the basis of their diet; ideally, they should be eaten at every meal.

CHAPTER 1:

BREAKFAST RECIPES

1. Amazing Almond & Banana Granola

Preparation Time: 5 minutes

Cooking Time: 70 minutes

Servings: 16

Ingredients:

- 2 peeled and chopped ripe bananas
- 8 cups of rolled oats
- 1 teaspoon of salt
- 2 cups of freshly pitted and chopped dates
- 1 cup of slivered and toasted almonds
- 1 teaspoon of almond extract

Directions:

1. Preheat the oven to 275o F.

2. Put a 13 x 18-inch baking sheets with parchment paper.

3. In a medium saucepan, add 1 cup of water and the dates, and bring to a boil. On medium heat, cook them for about 10 minutes. The dates will be soft and pulpy. Keep on adding water to the saucepan so that the dates do not stick to the pan.

4. After removing the dates from the heat, allow them to cool before you blend them with salt, almond extract, and bananas.

5. You will have a smooth and creamy puree.

6. Add this mixture to the oats and give it a thorough mix.

7. Divide the mixture into equal halves and spread over the baking sheets.

8. In your preheated oven, bake it for about 30-40 minutes, stirring every 10 minutes or so.

9. So that you will notice that granola is ready when it becomes crispy.

10. After removing the baking sheets from the oven, allow them to cool. Then add the slivered almonds.

11. You can store your granola in an airtight container and enjoy it whenever you are hungry.

Nutrition: Calories: 248.9 Fat 9.4 g Carbohydrate 35.9 g Protein 7.6 g

2. **Perfect Polenta with a Dose of Cranberries & Pears**

Preparation Time: 5 minutes

Cooking Time: 100 minutes

Servings: 4

Ingredients:

- 2 pears freshly cored, peeled, and diced
- 1 batch of warm basic polenta
- ¼ cup of brown rice syrup
- 1 teaspoon of ground cinnamon
- 1 cup of dried or fresh cranberries

Directions:

1. Warm the polenta in a medium-sized saucepan. Then add the cranberries, pears, and cinnamon powder.
2. Cook everything, stirring occasionally. You will know that the dish is ready when the pears are soft.
3. The entire dish will be done within 10 minutes.

4. Divide the polenta equally among 4 bowls. Add some pear compote as the last finishing touch.

5. Now you can dig into this hassle-free breakfast bowl full of goodness.

Nutrition: Calories: 185 Fat 4.6 g Protein 5 g Carbohydrate 6.1 g

3. Tempeh Bacon Smoked to Perfection

Preparation Time: 5 minutes

Cooking Time: 40 minutes

Servings: 10

Ingredients:

- 3 tablespoons of maple syrup
- 8-ounce packages of tempeh
- ¼ cup of soy or tamari sauce
- 2 teaspoons of liquid smoke

Directions:

1. In a steamer basket, steam the block of tempeh.
2. Put the tamari, maple syrup, and liquid smoke in a medium-sized bowl.
3. Once the tempeh cools down, slice into strips and add to the prepared marinade. Remember: the longer the tempeh marinates, the better the flavor will be. If possible, refrigerate overnight. If not, marinate for at least half an hour.

4. In a sauté pan, cook the tempeh on medium-high heat with a bit of the marinade.

5. Once the strips get crispy on one side, turn them over so that both sides are evenly cooked.

6. You can add some more marinade to cook the tempeh, but they should be properly caramelized. It will take about 5 minutes for each side to cook.

7. Enjoy the crispy caramelized tempeh with your favorite dip.

Nutrition: Calories: 130 Carbohydrate 17 g Protein 12 g Fat 1 g

4. **Vegan Muffins Breakfast Sandwich**

Preparation Time: 10 minutes

Cooking Time: 20 minutes

Servings: 2

Ingredients:

- Romesco Sauce: 3-4 tablespoons

- Fresh baby spinach: ½ cup

- Tofu Scramble: 2

- Vegan English muffins: 2

- Avocado: ½ peeled and sliced

- Sliced fresh tomato: 1

Directions:

1. In the oven, toast English muffin

2. Half the muffin and spread romesco sauce

3. Paste spinach to one side, tailed by avocado slices

4. Have warm tofu followed by a tomato slice

5. Place the other muffin half onto the preceding one

Nutrition: Carbs: 18g Protein: 12g Fats: 14g Calories: 276

5. Toasted Rye with Pumpkin Seed Butter

Preparation Time: 10 minutes

Cooking Time: 25 minutes and the cooling time

Servings: 4

Ingredients:

- Pumpkin seeds: 220g
- Date nectar: 1 tsp.
- Avocado oil: 2 tbsp.
- Rye bread: 4 slices toasted

Directions:

1. Toast the pumpkin seed on a frying pan on low heat for 5-7 minutes and stir in between
2. Let them turn golden and remove them from the pan
3. Add to the blender when they cool down and make fine powder
4. Add in avocado oil and salt and then again blend to form a paste
5. Add date nectars too and blend

6. On the toasted rye, spread one tablespoon of this butter and serve with your favorite toppings

Nutrition: Carbs: 3 g Protein: 5 g Fats: 10.3 g Calories: 127

6. Overnight Oats

Preparation Time: 15 minutes Cooking Time: 15 minutes plus overnight

Servings: 6

Ingredients:

- A pinch of Cinnamon
- 4 cups Almond milk
- 2 ½ cups Porridge oats
- 1 tbsp. Maple syrup
- 1 tbsp. Pumpkin seeds
- 1 tbsp. Chia seeds

Directions:

1. Add all the ingredients to the bowl and combine well
2. Cover the bowl and place it in the fridge overnight
3. Pour more milk in the morning
4. Serve with your favorite toppings

Nutrition Carbs: 32.3 g Protein: 10.2 g Fats: 12.7 g Calories: 298

7. Chickpeas Spread Sourdough Toast

Preparation Time: 15 minutes

Cooking Time: 15 minutes

Servings: 4

Ingredients

- 1 cup rinsed and drained chickpeas
- 1 cup pumpkin puree
- ½ cup vegan yogurt:
- Salt
- 4 slices toasted sourdough

Directions:

1. In a bowl add chickpeas and pumpkin puree and mash using a potato masher
2. Add in salt and yogurt and mix
3. Spread it on a toast and serve

Nutrition Carbs: 33.7g Protein: 8.45g Fats: 2.5g Calories: 187

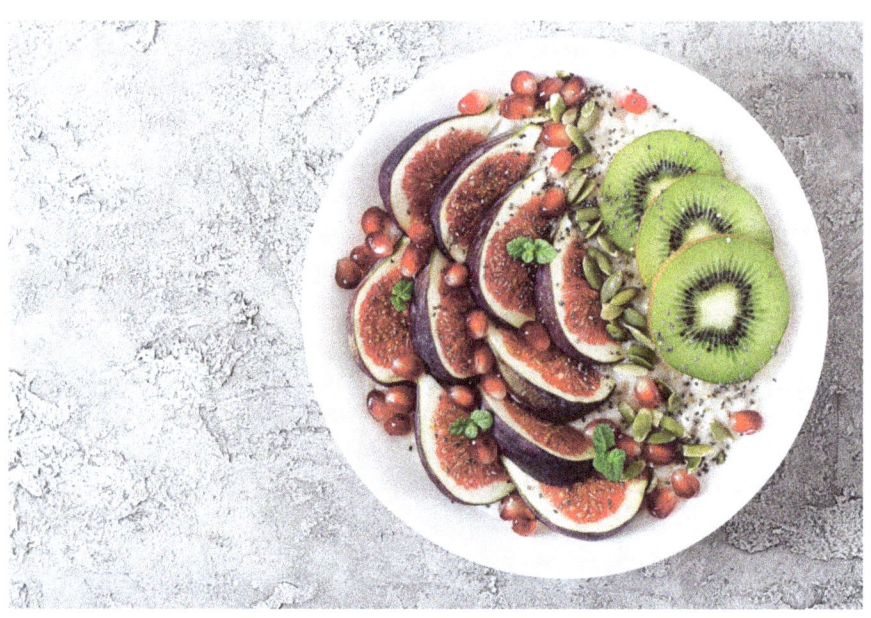
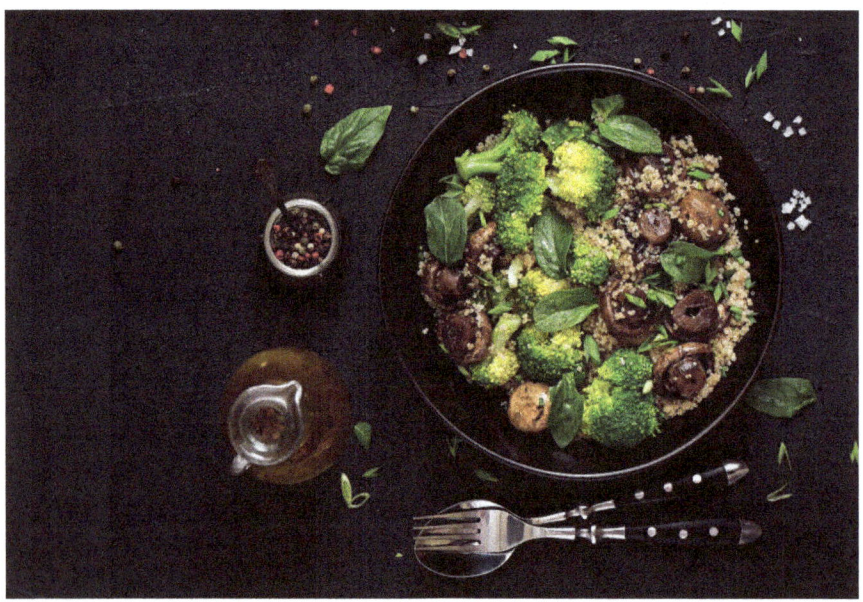

CHAPTER 2:

LUNCH RECIPES

8. Tomato Soup

Preparation Time: 10 minutes

Cooking Time: 8 hours

Servings: 6

Ingredients:

- 1 cup frozen mirepoix

- ⅓ Cup all-purpose flour

- 1 (28-ounce) can crushed tomatoes

- 1 (6-ounce) can tomato paste

- 1 tablespoon dried basil

- 1 teaspoon dried oregano

- 1 teaspoon salt, plus more for seasoning

- 4 cups chicken or vegetable broth

- 1 bay leaf

- 1 cup milk, warmed

- 2 tablespoons unsalted butter

- Freshly ground black pepper

- ⅔ Cup grated Parmesan cheese

Directions:

1. Combine the mirepoix, flour, crushed tomatoes, tomato paste, basil, oregano, and salt in the slow cooker. Whisk to stir your flour into the tomatoes to incorporate. Add the broth and stir. Add the bay leaf.

2. Cover your slow cooker for it to cook for 8 hours on low.

3. Discard the bay leaf. Stir in the warm milk and butter until the butter is melted. Season with salt and pepper, if needed.

4. Put the soup into your serving bowls, top each serving with Parmesan cheese, and serve.

Nutrition: Calories: 200 Fat: 8g Cholesterol: 22mg Carbohydrates: 25g Fiber: 6g Protein: 11g

9. Black Bean Soup

Preparation Time: 10 minutes

Cooking Time: 8 hours

Servings: 6

Ingredients:

- 8 ounces dried black beans
- 3½ cups water
- 1 smoked ham hock, rinsed
- 1 bay leaf
- 1 teaspoon dried oregano
- 1 teaspoon ground cumin
- 1 teaspoon garlic powder
- 1 teaspoon salt, plus more for seasoning
- Juice of 1 lime
- 1 (8-ounce) can tomato sauce
- Freshly ground black pepper

- Chopped fresh cilantro for garnish

Directions:

1. Combine the black beans, water, ham hock, bay leaf, oregano, cumin, garlic powder, and salt in your slow cooker.

2. Cover and wait for it to cook on low for 8 hours or until the beans are tender.

3. Discard the bay leaf. Stir in the lime juice and tomato sauce. Season with salt and pepper, if needed.

4. Serve your soup into bowls and garnish with cilantro.

Nutrition: Calories: 237 Total Fat: 7g Cholesterol: 43mg Carbohydrates: 23g Fiber: 6g Protein: 21g

10. French Onion Soup

Preparation Time: 15 minutes

Cooking Time: 8 hours

Servings: 4

Ingredients:

- 3 small yellow onions, cut into thin rings

- ¼ cup olive oil or canola oil

- Pinch salt

- Pinch freshly ground black pepper

- Pinch sugar

- 2 (13.5-ounce) cans beef consommé

- ½ cup water

- 4 slices crusty bread (French bread or a baguette works well)

- 1⅓ cups shredded Gruyère cheese

Directions:

1. Put the onions in the slow cooker. Add the olive oil, salt, pepper, and sugar and stir until the onions are coated.

2. Cover and wait for it to cook on low for 8 hours or until onions are soft and caramelized.

3. Pour in the consommé and water and turn the slow cooker to high. Cook until warmed through, about 10 minutes.

4. Put the top oven rack 6 inches below the broiler. Turn on the broiler.

5. Ladle the soup into four oven-safe bowls and place them on a rimmed baking sheet. Place a bread on top of each serving of soup. Sprinkle ⅓ cup of Gruyère cheese on top of each piece of bread.

6. Broil it for one to two minutes, or until the cheese is melted and starts to brown. Serve immediately.

Nutrition: Calories: 384 Total Fat: 24g Cholesterol: 33mg Sodium: 966mg Carbohydrates: 28g Fiber: 3g Protein: 17g

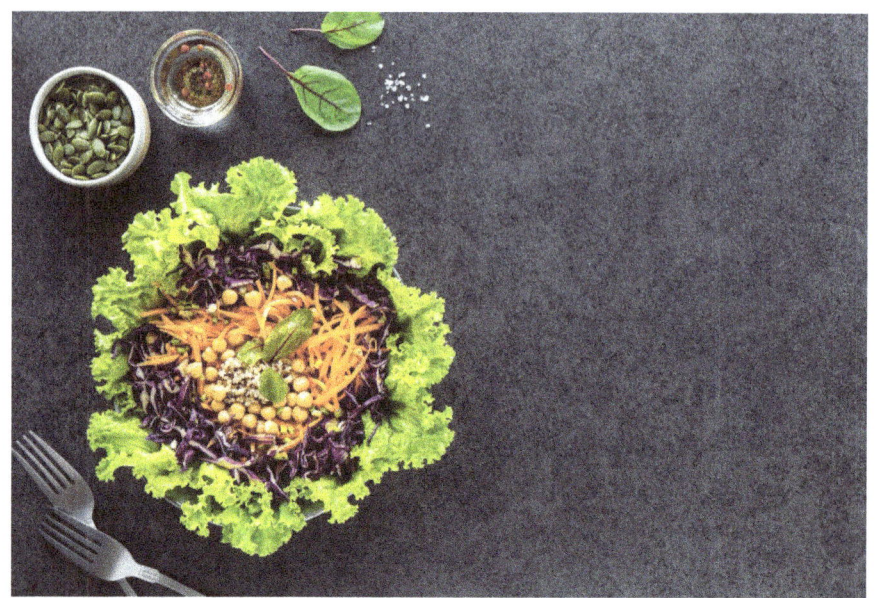

CHAPTER 3:

MAIN MEALS RECIPES

11. Stir Fry

Preparation Time: 10 minutes

Cooking Time: 15 minutes

Servings: 2

Ingredients:

- 3 cups chopped cabbage

- 1 large roughly chopped onion

- 2 roughly chopped green peppers - the veggies should add up to about 5 cups

- 3 tbsp. Chinese stir fry sauce

- 6 tbsp. water

- Olive oil for cooking

Directions:

1. Place olive oil in a wok over high heat. Sauté the onions for 2 minutes until soft and transparent. Add the cabbage and green peppers and cook for 7 - 10 minutes until everything is fully cooked.

2. Add the stir fry sauce and water. Toss the veggies lightly to make sure everything is covered.

3. Cook for another minute until the sauce becomes thick and glossy. Serve and enjoy!

Nutrition: Calories: 40 Carbs: 0g Fat: 4g Protein: 25g

12. Spanakorizo

Preparation Time: 5 minutes

Cooking Time: 20 minutes

Servings: 6

Ingredients:

- 1 ½ cup cooked brown rice
- 2 lb. fresh spinach
- 1 cup tomato sauce
- 2 chopped onions
- 1 cup water
- Olive oil for cooking

Directions:

1. Place olive oil in the large pot over high heat. Sauté the onions until soft and slightly transparent.

2. Add the fresh spinach, tomato sauce, and water and bring to a boil. Reduce the heat and add the rice.

3. Cover and let it simmer for 10 minutes.

4. Garnish with some fresh herbs and serve.

Nutrition: Calories: 295 Carbs: 48g Fat: 8g Protein: 10g

13. Roast Chili Lime Chickpeas

Preparation Time: 5 minutes Cooking Time: 30 minutes

Servings: 2

Ingredients:

- 1 15oz chickpeas, drained and rinsed
- 2 tablespoons olive oil
- 2 teaspoons chili powder
- 1 tablespoon lime zest
- ½ teaspoon salt

Directions:

1. Heat the oven to 400. Dry the drained chickpeas by patting them with a paper towel. Place the chickpeas into a bowl with the olive oil and toss them together well. Bake the chickpeas for thirty minutes on a baking sheet. After they have baked, place them back into the bowl and toss with the salt, lime zest, and chili powder.

Nutrition: Calories: 151 Carbs: 19g Fat: 6g Protein: 6g

14. Miso Spaghetti Squash

Preparation Time: 5 minutes

Cooking Time: 40 minutes

Servings: 4

Ingredients:

- 1 (3-pound) spaghetti squash
- 1 tablespoon hot water
- 1 tablespoon unseasoned rice vinegar
- 1 tablespoon white miso

Directions:

1. Preheat the oven to 400°F. Line a rimmed baking sheet with parchment paper.

2. Halve the squash lengthwise and place, cut-side down, on the prepared baking sheet. Bake for 35 to 40 minutes, until tender.

3. Cool until the squash is easy to handle. With a fork, scrape out the flesh, which will be stringy, like spaghetti. Transfer to a large bowl.

4. In a small bowl, combine the hot water, vinegar, and miso with a whisk or fork. Pour over the squash. Gently toss with tongs to coat the squash.

5. Divide the squash evenly among 4 single-serving containers. Let cool before sealing the lids.

Nutrition: Calories: 171 Carbs: 25g Fat: 2g Protein: 3g

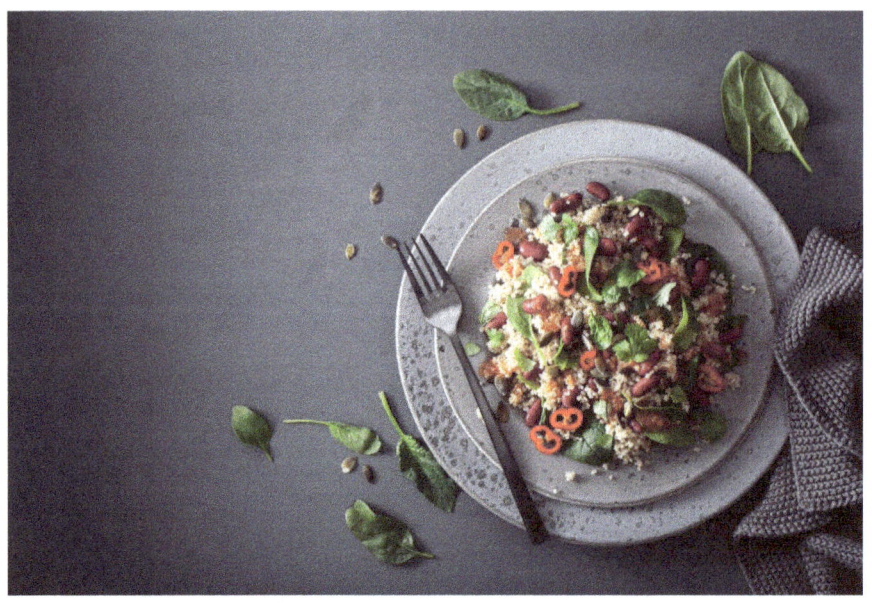

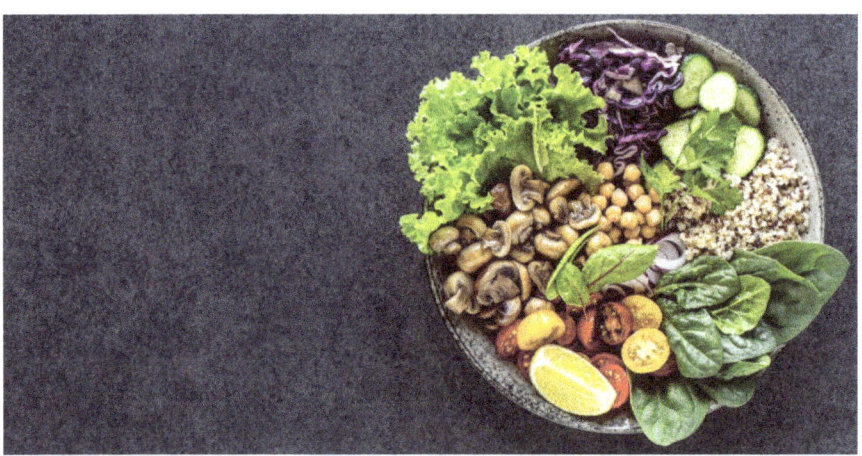

CHAPTER 4:

VEGETABLES, SALADS AND SIDES RECIPES

15. Mashed Cauliflower

Preparation Time: 10 minutes

Cooking Time: 15 minutes

Servings: 2

Ingredients:

- 4 cups cauliflower florets
- ¼ cup skim milk
- ¼ cup (2 ounces) grated Parmesan cheese
- 2 tablespoons butter

- 2 tablespoons extra-virgin olive oil

Directions:

- In a large pot over medium-high, cover the cauliflower with water and bring it to a boil.

- Reduce the heat to medium-low, cover, and simmer for about 10 minutes until the cauliflower is soft.

- Drain the cauliflower and return it to the pot. Add the milk, cheese, butter, olive oil, sea salt, and pepper.

- Using a potato masher, mash until smooth.

Nutrition:

Calories per Serving: 192;

Carbs: 16.1g;

Protein: 3.9g;

Fats: 13.8g

16. Broccoli with Ginger and Garlic

Preparation Time: 10 minutes

Cooking Time: 11 minutes

Servings: 2

Ingredients:

- 2 tablespoons extra-virgin olive oil
- 2 cups broccoli florets
- 1 tablespoon grated fresh ginger
- 3 garlic cloves, minced

Directions:

- In a large skillet over medium-high heat, heat the olive oil until it shimmers. Add the broccoli, ginger, sea salt, and pepper. Cook for about 10 minutes, stirring occasionally, until the broccoli is soft and starts to brown. Add the garlic and cook for 30 seconds, stirring constantly. Remove from the heat and serve.

Nutrition:

Calories per Serving: 192; Carbs: 16.1g; Protein: 3.9g; Fats: 13.8g

17. Balsamic Roasted Carrots

Preparation Time: 10 minutes Cooking Time: 30 minutes

Servings: 2

Ingredients:

- 1½ pounds carrots, quartered lengthwise
- 2 tablespoons extra-virgin olive oil
- ¼ teaspoon sea salt
- 1/8 teaspoon freshly ground black pepper
- 3 tablespoons balsamic vinegar

Directions:

- Preheat the oven to 425°F. In a large bowl, toss the carrots with the olive oil, sea salt, and pepper.
- Place in a single layer in a roasting pan or on a rimmed baking sheet. Roast for 20 to 30 minutes until the carrots are caramelized. Toss with the vinegar and serve.

Nutrition:

Calories per Serving: 192; Carbs: 16.1g; Protein: 3.9g; Fats: 13.8g

18. Chives and Radishes Platter

Preparation Time: 10 minutes

Cooking Time: 7 minutes

Servings: 2

Ingredients

- 2 cups radishes, quartered
- ½ cup vegetable stock
- Salt and pepper to taste
- 2 tablespoons melted ghee
- 1 tablespoon chives, chopped

Direction

- Add radishes, stock, salt, pepper, zest to your Ninja Foodi and stir Lock lid and cook on HIGH pressure for 7 minutes
- Quick release pressure. Add melted ghee, toss well. Sprinkle chives and enjoy!

Nutrition:

Calories per Serving: 192; Carbs: 16.1g; Protein: 3.9g; Fats: 13.8g

19. Healthy Rosemary and Celery Dish

Preparation Time: 10 minutes

Cooking Time: 5 minutes

Servings: 2

Ingredients

- 1-pound celery, cubed
- 1 cup of water
- 2 garlic cloves, minced
- Salt and pepper
- ¼ teaspoon dry rosemary
- 1 tablespoon olive oil

Direction

- Add water to your Ninja Foodi and place steamer basket
- Add celery cubs to basket and lock lid, cook on HIGH pressure for 4 minutes
- Quick release pressure. Take a bowl and add mix in oil, garlic, and rosemary. Whisk well

- Add steamed celery to the bowl and toss well, spread on a lined baking sheet

- Broil for 3 minutes using the Air Crisping lid at 250 degrees F. Serve and enjoy!

Nutrition:

Calories: 190,

Fats: 10g,

Dietary Fiber: 3.1g,

Carbohydrates: 25.5g,

Protein: 3.2g

20. Hearty Cheesy Cauliflower

Time: 10 minutes Cooking Time: 35 minutes   Servings: 2

Ingredients

- 1 tablespoon Keto-Friendly mustard
- 1 head cauliflower
- 1 teaspoon avocado mayonnaise
- ½ cup parmesan cheese, grated
- ¼ cup butter, cut into small pieces

Directions

- Set your Ninja Foodi to Sauté mode and add butter, let it melt
- Add cauliflower and Sauté for 3 minutes Add rest of the ingredients and lock lid, cook on HIGH pressure for 30 minutes
- Release pressure naturally over 10 minutes. Serve and enjoy!

Nutrition:

Calories: 190, Fats: 10g, Dietary Fiber: 3.1g, Carbohydrates: 25.5g, Protein: 3.2g

21. Mesmerizing Spinach Quiche

Preparation Time: 10 minutes

Cooking Time: 33 minutes

Servings: 2

Ingredients

- 1 tablespoon butter, melted
- 1 pack (10 ounces) frozen spinach, thawed
- 5 organic eggs, beaten
- Salt and pepper to taste
- 3 cups Monterey Jack Cheese, shredded

Directions

- Set your Ninja Foodi to Sauté mode and let it heat up, add butter and let the butter melt
- Add spinach and Sauté for 3 minutes, transfer the Sautéed spinach to a bowl
- Add eggs, cheese, salt, and pepper to a bowl and mix it well

- Transfer the mixture to greased quiche molds and transfer the mold to your Foodi

- Close the lid and choose the "Bake/Roast" mode and let it cook for 30 minutes at 360 degrees F. Once done, open lid and transfer the dish out

- Cut into wedges and serve. Enjoy!

Nutrition:

Calories per Serving: 192;

Carbs: 16.1g;

Protein: 3.9g;

Fats: 13.8g

22. Simple Mushroom Hats and Eggs

Preparation Time: 10 minutes

Cooking Time: 9 minutes

Servings: 2

Ingredients

- 4 ounces mushroom hats
- 1 teaspoon butter, melted
- 4 quail eggs
- ½ teaspoon ground black pepper
- ¼ teaspoon salt

Directions

- Spread the mushroom hats with the butter inside. Then beat the eggs into mushroom hats
- Sprinkle with salt and ground black pepper. Transfer the mushroom hats on the rack
- Lower the air fryer lid. Cook the meat for 7 minutes at 365 F

- Check the mushroom, if it is not cooked fully then cook them for 2 minutes more

- Serve and enjoy!

Nutrition:

Calories: 190,

Fats: 10g,

Dietary Fiber: 3.1g,

Carbohydrates: 25.5g,

Protein: 3.2g

CHAPTER 5:

DESSERT RECIPES

23. Salted Caramel Coconut Balls

Preparation Time: 15 minutes

Cooking Time: 25 minutes

Servings: 12 balls

Ingredients:

- 1 cup pitted dates
- 1 cup almonds
- ¼ cup coconut flakes
- ¼ tsp. salt

Directions:

1. Blend the dates, almonds, and salt until a sticky dough forms in your food processor.

2. Divide dough into 12. Roll this to make balls. Roll the balls in the coconut flakes, making sure they're completely covered, and serve.

Nutrition: Calories: 33 Total fat: 3g Carbohydrates: 1g Protein: 0g

24. Baked Pears

Preparation Time: 5 minutes

Cooking Time: 25 minutes

Servings: 2

Ingredients:

- 2 halved pears
- 1 tsp dark syrup
- Cinnamon

Directions:

1. Preheat the oven to 350 F.
2. Scoop the seeds out of your pears and place them in your baking tray. Drizzle with syrup and sprinkle with cinnamon.
3. Bake for 20 - 25 minutes and serve while warm.

Nutrition: Calories: 208 Total fat: 498g Carbohydrates: 3g Protein: 0g

25. Chocolate Mousse

Preparation Time: 15 minutes

Cooking Time: 0 minutes

Servings: 6

Ingredients:

- 150 g chocolate
- 2 ripe avocados
- 5 oz. coconut cream
- 3 tbsps. dark syrup
- 2 tbsps. cocoa powder

Directions:

1. Melt the chocolate using the Bunsen burner method. Remove the bowl from the heat and let cool slightly.

2. Place your avocados, coconut cream, syrup, and cocoa powder and pulse until everything is blended.

3. Add chocolate and pulse all over again until the mixture is creamy and smooth.

4. Divide mixture into six small bowls and chill in the refrigerator for 30 minutes.

5. Garnish with grated chocolate and serve.

Nutrition: Calories: 49 Total fat: 10g Carbohydrates: 2g Protein: 2g

26. Super Tea Spiced Poached Pears

Preparation Time: 10 minutes

Cooking Time: 4 hours and 5 minutes

Servings: 4

Ingredients:

- 4 medium-sized pears, peeled
- 1 tablespoon of grated ginger
- 5 cardamom pods
- 1 cinnamon stick, split in half
- 1/4 cup of maple syrup
- 16 fluid ounce of orange juice

Directions:

1. Cut off the bottom of each pear and centralize it.
2. Using a 4 quarts slow cooker, place the pears in an upright position, and add the remaining ingredients.

3. Cover the top, plug in the slow cooker; adjust the cooking time to 4 hours and let it cook on the high heat setting or until it gets soft.

4. Sprinkle it with the ground cinnamon over each pear, top it with the nuts and serve.

Nutrition: Calories: 98 Carbohydrates: 26g Protein: 1g Fats: 0g

27. Warming Baked Apples

Preparation Time: 10 minutes

Cooking Time: 2 hours and 10 minutes

Servings: 5

Ingredients:

- 4 medium-sized apples
- 1/2 cup of granola
- 4 teaspoon of maple syrup
- 2 tablespoons of melted vegan butter, unsalted

Directions:

1. Cut off the top of the apple and remove the core from each apple using a measuring spoon.
2. Fill the center of each apple with 1/8 cup of granola and place it in a 4-quarts slow cooker.
3. Drizzle with butter and then sprinkle with a teaspoon maple syrup over each apple.

4. Cover the top, plug in the slow cooker; adjust the cooking time to 2 hours and let it cook on the high heat setting or until it gets tender.

5. Serve right away.

Nutrition: Calories: 162 Carbohydrates: 42g Protein: 0.5g Fats: 0.3g

CHAPTER 6:

SNACK RECIPES

28. Lemon and Olive Pasta

Preparation Time: 5 minutes

Cooking Time: 7-8 minutes

Servings: 2

Ingredients:

- 1 Vidalia onion, diced

- 2 garlic cloves, minced

- 1 tablespoon olive oil

- 3½ cups water or unsalted vegetable broth

- 10 ounces bow ties, small shells, or other small pasta (about 3¾ cups)

- Grated zest and juice of 1 lemon

- ¼ cup pitted black olives, chopped

- Salt

- Freshly ground black pepper

Directions:

1. On your electric pressure cooker, select Sauté. Add the onion, garlic, and olive oil. Cook for 7 to 8 minutes, stir until the onion is lightly browned.
2. Add the water and pasta. Cancel Sauté.
3. Close and lock lid, then ensure the pressure valve is sealed, then select High Pressure and set the time for 4 minutes.
4. Once cooked, quickly release the pressure, being careful not to get your fingers or face near the steam release.
5. Once done, carefully unlock, then remove the lid. Stir the pasta and drain any excess water. Stir in the lemon zest and juice and the olives. Taste and add more olive oil and season with salt and pepper.

Nutrition: Calories: 414 Total fat: 7g Protein: 15g Sodium: 436mg Fiber: 9g

29. Cheesy Macaroni

Preparation Time: 10 minutes

Cooking Time: 5 minutes

Servings: 4

Ingredients:

- 1 pound macaroni or other small pasta
- 5½ cups water, divided
- ½ to 1 teaspoon salt, plus more as needed
- 2 yellow potatoes or red potatoes, peeled and cut into chunks
- 2 carrots, cut into chunks (of similar size to the potatoes)
- ½ cup nondairy milk
- ¼ cup nutritional yeast
- 1 tablespoon freshly squeezed lemon juice
- 2 teaspoons onion powder
- 1 teaspoon garlic powder
- Pinch red pepper flakes or cayenne (optional)

Directions:

1. Using an electric pressure cooker pot, combine the macaroni, 4 cups of water, and a pinch of salt.

2. Place trivet in a pot and put potatoes and carrots in a steaming basket on top of the trivet. Close and lock the lid to ensure the pressure valve is sealed. Select high pressure, then set the time for 5 minutes.

3. Once done, release the pressure carefully not to get your fingers or face near the steam release.

4. Once done, remove the lid and carefully pull out the steaming basket with the potatoes and carrots. Transfer it to a blender, then add the milk, remaining 1½ cups of water, salt, nutritional yeast, lemon juice, red pepper flakes (if using), onion powder, and garlic powder. Purée until smooth. Stir the cheese sauce into the macaroni. Taste and season with more salt or other seasonings, if needed.

Nutrition: Calories: 501 Total fat: 3g Protein: 23g Sodium: 346mg Fiber: 14g

30. Creamy Mushroom Rigatoni

Preparation Time: 10 minutes Cooking Time: 7-8 minutes

Servings: 4

Ingredients:

- 12 ounce mushrooms, sliced (about 5 cups)
- 2 to 3 teaspoons olive oil
- 3 cups water or unsalted vegetable broth
- ¼ to ½ teaspoon salt, plus more as needed
- 12 ounces rigatoni (about 4½ cups)
- 1 cup unsweetened nondairy milk
- 2 tablespoons nutritional yeast
- 1 tablespoon dried oregano
- 1 teaspoon onion powder
- ½ teaspoon garlic powder
- ¼ teaspoon ground nutmeg (optional)
- Freshly ground black pepper

Directions:

1. On your electric pressure cooker, select Sauté. Add the mushrooms and olive oil and cook for 7 to 8 minutes, stirring occasionally, until the mushrooms are lightly browned. Cancel Sauté.

2. Add the water, salt, and pasta. Close and lock the lid to ensure the pressure valve is sealed, then set the time for 3 minutes in high pressure.

3. Once complete, release pressure naturally for 5 minutes. Quickly release any remaining pressure. Make sure to carefully release.

4. Once done and the pressure is released, remove the lid carefully. Drain off any excess water and stir in the milk, nutritional yeast, oregano, onion powder, garlic powder, and nutmeg (if using). To taste, season it with salt and pepper if needed. You may have to pull apart any noodles that have stuck together.

5. On the pressure cooker, select Sauté or Simmer. Cook for 2 to 3 minutes and stir occasionally until the sauce thickens slightly.

Nutrition: Calories: 506 Total fat: 6g Protein: 23g; Sodium: 200mg Fiber: 12g

31. Southwest Pasta

Preparation Time: 5 minutes Cooking Time: 5-6 minutes

Servings: 4

Ingredients:

- 1 red onion, diced
- 1 to 2 teaspoons olive oil
- 1 to 2 teaspoons ground chipotle pepper
- 1 (28-ounce) can crushed tomatoes
- 8 ounces rotini, fusilli, or penne
- 1 cup water or unsalted vegetable broth
- 1½ cups fresh or frozen corn
- 1½ cups cooked black beans (from ½ cup dried)
- Salt
- Freshly ground black pepper

Directions: On your electric pressure cooker, select Sauté. Add the red onion and olive oil and cook for 5 to 6 minutes, stirring occasionally, until the onion is lightly browned. Cancel Sauté.

1. Stir in the chipotle pepper, tomatoes, pasta, and water. Make sure lock the lid and the pressure valve is sealed. Select high pressure and set it for 4 minutes.

2. Once cooking is complete, let the pressure release naturally for 4 minutes. Carefully release the remaining pressure. Be careful in using this.

3. Once done and the pressure is released, remove the lid carefully. Stir in the corn and black beans to warm. Taste and season with salt and pepper.

Nutrition: Calories: 366 Total fat: 4 Protein: 17g Sodium: 176mg Fiber: 14g

32. Peanut Noodles

Preparation Time: 10 minutes Cooking Time: 2 minutes

Servings: 4

Ingredients:

- ½ cup smooth peanut butter
- ¼ cup tamari or soy sauce
- ¼ cup rice vinegar or apple cider vinegar
- 1 to 2 tablespoons toasted sesame oil (optional)
- 1 teaspoon ground ginger (optional)
- Pinch red pepper flakes or cayenne (optional)
- 2½ cups water, plus more as needed
- 8 ounces thick udon noodles or soba noodles
- 4 carrots, cut into matchsticks
- ½ head broccoli, cut into 1-inch pieces

Directions: Stir together the peanut butter, tamari, vinegar, sesame oil (if using), ginger (if using), and red pepper flakes (if using) until smooth and combined in a small bowl.

1. Pour the peanut sauce into your electric pressure cooker's cooking pot. Add the water.

2. Add the noodles to the pot, breaking them into shorter strands if they're too long to lie flat on the bottom and making sure the liquid covers them. Add another ¼ cup of water if needed. Stir the noodles a bit to make sure they don't stick together.

3. Lay the carrots and then the broccoli on top, or put them in a steaming basket on top of a trivet. Close and lock the lid to ensure the pressure valve is sealed. Select Low Pressure and set the time for 2 minutes.

4. When cooking time is complete, make sure to quickly release the pressure, and be careful.

5. Once done and the pressure is released, remove the lid carefully. Toss everything together, breaking up any noodles that may have stuck together, and serve.

Nutrition: Calories: 467 Total fat: 20g Protein: 20g Sodium: 1.5mg Fiber: 5g

33. Red Curry Noodles

Preparation Time: 5 minutes

Cooking Time: 10 minutes

Servings: 4

Ingredients:

- 2 cups water
- 1 (13.5-ounce) can coconut milk
- ¼ cup red curry paste
- 1 tablespoon freshly squeezed lime juice
- 1 tablespoon tamari or soy sauce
- 1 to 2 teaspoons toasted sesame oil
- 8 ounces thick ramen noodles or wide brown rice noodles

Directions:

1. Using an electric pressure cooker, combine water, coconut milk, curry paste, lime juice, tamari, and sesame oil. Add the noodles, breaking them into shorter strands if they're too long to lie flat on the bottom. Close and lock the lid to ensure the pressure

valve is sealed. Select then the high pressure and set it for 1 minute.

2. Once done cooking, remove the lid carefully until pressure is released. Toss everything together, breaking up any noodles that may have stuck together, and serve.

3. Serving tip: Top these yummy noodles with chopped veggies, and pair with greens sautéed in sesame oil.

Nutrition: Calories: 611 Total fat: 36g Protein: 6g Sodium: 473mg Fiber: 2g

34. Sun-Dried Tomato Pasta

Preparation Time: 10 minutes

Cooking Time: 20 minutes

Servings: 4

Ingredients:

- 1 large Vidalia onion, diced
- 1 teaspoon olive oil, plus more for finishing
- 10 ounces (about 3 cups) penne, rotini, or fusilli
- ¼ cup sun-dried tomatoes, chopped
- 2 cups water or unsalted vegetable broth
- ½ teaspoon salt, plus more as needed
- 2 tablespoons finely chopped fresh basil
- 1 cup cherry tomatoes, halved or quartered
- ½ teaspoon garlic powder (optional)
- Freshly ground black pepper

Directions:

1. On your electric pressure cooker, select Sauté. Add the onion and olive oil and cook for 4 to 5 minutes, stirring occasionally, until the onion is softened.

2. Add the pasta, sun-dried tomatoes, water, and a pinch of salt. Cancel Sauté.

3. Close then lock the lid. Ensure that it is safe, then select high pressure. After, set it for 4 minutes.

4. Once done, release the pressure slowly for 5 minutes. Then release any remaining pressure. Make sure to do some extra precautionary when using a pressure cooker.

5. Once done and the pressure is released, remove the lid carefully. Select Sauté or Simmer. Toss in the basil, cherry tomatoes, garlic powder (if using), and another drizzle of olive oil. Add more salt, if needed, and pepper.

Nutrition: Calories: 343 Total fat: 3g Protein: 14g Sodium: 300mg Fiber: 9g

CHAPTER 7:

JUICES AND SMOOTHIES RECIPES

35. Beet and Orange Smoothie

Preparation time: 5 minutes

Cooking time: 0 minutes

Servings: 1

Ingredients:

- 1 Cup chopped zucchini rounds, frozen
- 1 cup spinach
- 1 small peeled navel orange, frozen
- 1 small chopped beet

- 1 scoop of vanilla protein powder

- 1 cup almond milk, unsweetened

Directions:

1. Place all the ingredients in the order in a food processor or blender and then pulse for 2 to 3 minutes at high speed until smooth.

2. Pour the smoothie into a glass and then serve.

Nutrition: Calories: 253 Cal Fat: 5 g Carbs: 44.6 g Protein: 3 g

36. Strawberry, Banana, and Coconut Shake

Preparation time: 5 minutes

Cooking time: 0 minutes

Servings: 1

Ingredients:

- 1 tablespoon coconut flakes
- 1/2 cups frozen banana slices
- 1 strawberries, sliced
- 1/2 cup coconut milk, unsweetened
- 1/4 cup strawberries for topping

Directions:

1. Place all the ingredients in the order in a food processor or blender, except for topping, and then pulse for 2 to 3 minutes at high speed until smooth.
2. Pour the smoothie into a glass and then serve.

Nutrition: Calories: 335 Fat: 5 g Carbs: 75 g Protein: 4 g

37. Green Colada

Preparation time: 5 minutes

Cooking time: 0 minutes

Servings: 1

Ingredients:

- 1/2 cup frozen pineapple chunks
- 1/2 banana
- 1/2 teaspoon spirulina powder
- 1/4 teaspoon vanilla extract, unsweetened
- 1 cup of coconut milk

Directions:

1. Place all the ingredients in the order in a food processor or blender and then pulse for 2 to 3 minutes at high speed until smooth.
2. Pour the smoothie into a glass and then serve.

Nutrition: Calories: 127 Fat: 3 g Carbs: 25 g Protein: 3 g

38. Avocado Spinach Smoothie

Preparation Time: 5 minutes

Cooking Time: 5 minutes

Servings: 2

Ingredients

- Coconut milk: 1 cup
- Frozen banana: 1 small sliced
- Avocado: 1 small
- Baby spinach: 1 ½ cup

Directions:

1. Add all the ingredients to the blender
2. Blend to form a smooth consistency

Nutrition Carbs: 29.2 g Protein: 9.2 g Fats: 10.3 g Calories: 235

39. Almond Spinach Smoothie

Preparation Time: 15 minutes

Cooking Time: 5 minutes

Servings: 1

Ingredients

- Large banana: 1
- Ice cubes: 4
- Almonds: ¼ cup
- Fresh spinach: 1 cup
- Rolled oats: 2 tbsp.
- Unsweetened almond milk: ¾ cup

Directions:

1. Add all the ingredients to the blender
2. Blend to form a smooth consistency

Nutrition Carbs: 49.2 g Protein: 11.9 g Fats: 19.9 g Calories: 406

40. 3-Ingredient Mango Smoothie

Preparation Time: 15 minutes

Cooking Time: 5 minutes

Servings: 1

Ingredients

- Frozen mango chunks: 1 cup
- Oat milk: ½ cup
- Frozen banana: 1 large sliced

Directions:

1. Add all the ingredients to the blender
2. Blend until smooth

Nutrition Carbs: 67.1 g Protein: 3.5 g Fats: 1.7 g Calories: 276

CHAPTER 8:

OTHER RECIPES

41. Tahini Miso Dressing

Preparation Time: 10 minutes Cooking Time: 0 minutes

Servings: 2

Ingredients:

- ¼ cup tahini
- 1 tablespoon tamari or low-sodium soy sauce
- 1 tablespoon white miso
- 1 tablespoon freshly squeezed lemon juice
- 1 tablespoon maple syrup or honey
- ¼ cup warm water
- Freshly ground black pepper

Directions:

1. In a small bowl, whisk the tahini, tamari, miso, lemon juice, and maple syrup together. Whisk in the water and black pepper. Store in an airtight container in the refrigerator for up to six months.

Nutrition: Calories: 76 Fat: 6g Carbs: 5g Protein: 2g

42. Balsamic Roasted Tomatoes

Preparation Time: 10 minutes

Cooking Time: 4 hours

Servings: 6

Ingredients:

- 6 medium tomatoes or 1 pint cherry tomatoes
- ¼ cup, plus 1 tablespoon olive oil
- Kosher salt
- Freshly ground black pepper
- 2 teaspoons balsamic vinegar

Directions:

1. Preheat the oven to 300°F. Put your rimmed baking sheet with parchment paper.
2. Wash and dry the tomatoes, and halve them crosswise. Put them cut-side up on the parchment paper, and drizzle them with ¼ cup of olive oil, allowing the oil to pool on the parchment paper. Sprinkle with salt and pepper.

3. Roast for 3 to 4 hours, or until the edges of the tomatoes are puckered, and the cut surface is a little dry.

4. Sprinkle with the balsamic vinegar and let cool on the baking sheet.

5. Pack into an airtight container and pour any excess oil from the parchment paper on top. Add the remaining 1 tablespoon of oil to the container. Seal and refrigerate for up to one month.

Nutrition: Calories: 123 Fat: 12g Carbs: 5g Protein: 1g

43. Crispy Spicy Chickpeas

Preparation Time: 5 minutes

Cooking Time: 30 minutes

Servings: 1

Ingredients:

- 1 cup canned chickpeas, drained and rinsed
- 1 tablespoon olive oil
- ½ teaspoon kosher salt
- ⅛ Teaspoon freshly ground black pepper
- ½ teaspoon smoked paprika
- ⅛ Teaspoon cayenne pepper

Directions:

1. Preheat the oven to 400°F.
2. Remove any remaining moisture from the chickpeas by rolling them between two paper towels. Place in a medium bowl.
3. Add the olive oil, salt, and pepper to the bowl and toss to completely coat the chickpeas.

4. Spread them out on a baking sheet. Roast for 20 minutes, stir, and roast for an additional 10 minutes, or until lightly crisped.

5. When it's still warm, toss the chickpeas with the smoked paprika and cayenne pepper. Adding the spices last prevents them from charring in the oven and provides a crispier chickpea.

6. You can keep it at room temperature in an open container for several days. This keeps them crisper longer, although they'll start to lose some crispness over time. They can also be stored in the refrigerator once they've completely cooled.

Nutrition: Calories: 101 Fat: 4g Carbs: 14g Protein: 3g

44. Roasted Pumpkin Seeds

Preparation Time: 5 minutes Cooking Time: 10 minutes

Servings: 1

Ingredients:

- 1 cup unsalted pumpkin seeds

- 1 teaspoon olive oil

- ¼ teaspoon kosher salt

- Pinch cayenne pepper

- Pinch smoked paprika

Directions:

1. Using a small bowl, combine all of the ingredients.

2. Heat a small sauté pan over medium-low heat. Add the pumpkin seeds and sauté, tossing frequently as they brown, for 10 minutes, or until they reach your preferred level of toasting.

3. Cool and store at room temperature in an airtight container for up to two months or in the refrigerator for up to one year.

Nutrition: Calories: 20 Fat: 1g Carbs: 2g Protein: 1g

45. Lemony Breadcrumbs

Preparation Time: 5 minutes

Cooking Time: 10 minutes

Servings: 1

Ingredients:

- 2 teaspoons olive oil
- 1 cup panko
- ⅛ Teaspoon kosher salt
- ⅛ Teaspoon freshly ground black pepper
- Zest of 1 lemon (about ½ teaspoon or more, to taste)

Directions:

1. Using a small skillet over a medium heat, warm the olive oil. Add the panko, salt, and pepper. Toss to lightly coat and toast until the breadcrumbs are a golden color, about 3 minutes. You'll need to stir the breadcrumbs about every 30 seconds, so they toast evenly.

2. Take it out from the heat and stir in the lemon zest.

3. Transfer to a plate to cool before storing in an airtight container.

Nutrition: Calories: 63 Fat: 2g Carbs: 10g Protein: 2g

46. Cauliflower Skillet Steaks

Preparation Time: 15 minutes

Cooking Time: 15 minutes

Servings: 4

Ingredients:

- 1 large head cauliflower, sliced into 6 (1-inch-thick) steaks
- 2 tablespoons olive oil, divided
- ½ teaspoon smoked paprika
- ½ teaspoon kosher salt
- ¼ teaspoon cayenne pepper
- Balsamic Roasted Tomatoes

Directions:

1. Rub both sides of the cauliflower steaks lightly with 1 tablespoon of olive oil, and sprinkle on both sides with the paprika, salt, and cayenne.
2. Heat the remaining 1 tablespoon of olive oil in a large sauté pan over medium-high heat. Arrange the cauliflower steaks in the

pan, including any extra florets. You need to cook the steaks in two batches.

3. Cook the cauliflower until slightly crisped, about 3 minutes per side. Reduce the heat to medium and continue to cook for another 8 to 10 minutes, or until the cauliflower is tender when pierced with a sharp knife.

4. Serve the cauliflower steaks topped with the roasted tomatoes.

Nutrition: Calories: 114 Fat: 8g Carbs: 11g Protein: 4g

47. Lemony Kale, Avocado, And Chickpea Salad

Preparation Time: 20 minutes

Cooking Time: 0 minutes

Servings: 4

Ingredients:

- 1 avocado, halved
- 2 tablespoons freshly squeezed lemon juice, divided
- ½ teaspoon kosher salt, divided
- 1 bunch curly kale, stems removed and discarded, leaves coarsely chopped (about 8 cups)
- 1 (15-ounce) can chickpeas, drained and rinsed
- 2 tablespoons extra-virgin olive oil
- ¼ teaspoon freshly ground black pepper
- ¼ cup Roasted Pumpkin Seeds or store-bought

Direction:

1. Slice your avocado, then coop its flesh from one of the avocado halves out of its skin and put it in a large bowl. Put a 1

tablespoon of lemon juice and ¼ teaspoon of salt and mash everything together. Add the coarsely chopped kale leaves and massage them by hand with the avocado mash until the kale becomes tender. Place the kale-avocado mash on a serving plate.

2. Remove the flesh of the remaining avocado half from its skin and chop into bite-size chunks. Place in the bowl that contained the kale and add the chickpeas.

3. In a small bowl, whisk together the olive oil, the remaining 1 tablespoon of lemon juice, the remaining ¼ teaspoon of salt, and the pepper. Drizzle over the chickpeas and avocado and toss to combine. Pile on top of the kale-avocado mash and top with the roasted pumpkin seeds.

Nutrition: Calories: 383 Fat: 20g Carbs: 43g Protein: 14g

48. Lentil Potato Salad

Preparation Time: 10 minutes

Cooking Time: 25 minutes

Servings: 2

Ingredients:

- ½ cup beluga lentils
- 8 fingerling potatoes
- 1 cup thinly sliced scallions
- ¼ cup halved cherry tomatoes
- ¼ cup Lemon Vinaigrette
- Kosher salt, to taste
- Freshly ground black pepper, to taste

Directions:

1. Pour 2 cups of water to simmer in a small pot and add the lentils. Cover and simmer for 20 to 25 minutes, or until the lentils are tender. Drain and set aside to cool.

2. While the lentils are cooking, bring a medium pot of well-salted water to a boil and add the potatoes. Low heat to simmer and cook for about 15 minutes, or until the potatoes are tender. Drain. Once cool enough to handle, slice, or halve the potatoes.

3. Place the lentils on a serving plate and top with the potatoes, scallions, and tomatoes. Drizzle with the vinaigrette and season with salt and pepper.

Nutrition: Calories: 400 Fat: 26g Carbs: 39g Protein: 7g

49. Curried Apple Chips

Preparation Time: 15 minutes

Cooking Time: 1 hour and 30 minutes

Servings: 25 chips

Ingredients:

- 1 tablespoon freshly squeezed lemon juice
- ½ cup water
- 2 apples, such as Fuji or Honey crisp, cored and thinly sliced into rings
- 1 teaspoon curry powder

Directions:

1. Preheat the oven to 200°F. Put a rimmed baking sheet with parchment paper.
2. Mix the lemon juice and water together in a medium bowl. As soon as the apples are sliced, add them to the bowl to soak for 2 minutes. Drain and pat dry with paper towels. Arrange in a single layer on the baking sheet.

3. Place the curry powder in a sieve or other sifter and lightly sprinkle the apple slices. Not too much curry goes a long way, so it's okay not to dust both sides of the apple rings.

4. In you preheated oven, bake it for 45 minutes. After 45 minutes, turn the slices over and bake for another 45 minutes, again without opening the oven. If you find the apple chips need additional crisping, bake for another 15 minutes.

5. For the crispiest texture, let the chips cool before eating, but they're pretty fabulous slightly warm.

Nutrition: Calories: 61 Fat: 0g Carbs: 16g Protein: 0g

50. Bok Choy–Asparagus Salad

Preparation Time: 20 minutes

Cooking Time: 0 minutes

Servings: 4

Ingredients:

- 4 cups coarsely chopped baby bok Choy
- 1½ cups asparagus, trimmed and cut into 1½-inch lengths
- 1 cup cauliflower rice
- 1 cup strawberries, chopped into bite-size chunks
- 1 mango, peeled and diced
- ½ cup scallions, sliced into 1-inch lengths
- ¼ cup Lemon Vinaigrette

Directions:

1. In a large bowl, combine the bok choy, asparagus, cauliflower rice, strawberries, mango, and scallions. Drizzle with the vinaigrette and gently toss.

Nutrition: Calories: 210 Fat: 14g Carbs: 21g Protein: 3g

CONCLUSION

Well done! Thank you for reaching the end of this book, The Complete Vegetarian Cookbook.

Hopefully, this book has helped you understand that making vegetarian recipes and diet easier can improve your life, not only by improving your health and helping you lose weight, but also by saving you money and time.

Remember that vegetarianism is a choice, not a religion.

Be flexible when it comes to your diet and enjoy new tastes and experiences.

The best tip I can give you about making vegetarian recipes is to experiment and have fun!

Here are some more tips to help you with your vegetarian diet:

1. Remember that vegetarianism is not a destination, it is a journey.

2. A vegetarian diet is plant-based. This means that you should try to eat more plants and less animal products. You should also be careful not to replace whole foods with their processed counterparts, such as replacing whole foods such as fruits and vegetables with fruit juice and pasta sauce.

3. Try to avoid processed food whenever possible, while still maintaining your balanced diet and nutrients that you need for your health. An easier way of doing this will be to make your own food when possible and try to avoid packaged, pre-prepared foods at the grocery store.

4. Avoid processed food products that contain artificial ingredients, such as sweeteners, colors, and flavors.

5. Avoid highly processed meat substitutes. Remember to use meat substitutes in moderation or as an occasional treat.

6. If you choose to eat meat substitutes such as tofu, be sure to thoroughly cook it and try different ways of preparing it

7. You may need to gradually introduce your family and friends to your new eating habits. Don't expect everyone to support you or enjoy the same things you do when it comes to vegetarian recipes. As long as you are happy with your food choices, that is the most important thing – even if it means making some changes at home!

When you are having a hard time, always remember this: You can always choose to stop being a vegetarian.

You can simply start eating meat again if you are struggling with your new diet.

Remember that it is okay to be a part-time vegetarian, but if you find that you cannot maintain the lifestyle or are unhappy with your choice, it is always better to go back to eating a non-veg diet.

There is no shame in making changes to your vegetarian recipe routine if you need to, and you will not shame yourself for deciding that a strict vegetarian diet does not work for you.

I know that there are many books and choosing my book is amazing. I am thankful that you stopped and took the time to decide. You made a great decision, and I am sure that you enjoyed it.

I will be even happier if you will add some comments. Feedbacks helped by growing, and they still do. They help me to choose better content and new ideas. So, maybe your feedback can trigger an idea for my next book. Thank you again for downloading this book!

I hope you enjoyed reading my book!

www.ingramcontent.com/pod-product-compliance
Lightning Source LLC
Chambersburg PA
CBHW070937080526
44589CB00013B/1543